HOW TO PUT INSOMNIA TO SLEEP

Learn how to get to sleep fast and stay asleep without using drugs or alcohol - and get back to sleep if you should wake up - using techniques from NLP, self hypnosis and meditation

BY

ABBY EAGLE

Published by Abby Eagle

PO Box 902 Palm Beach
Qld 4221 Australia
www.abbyeagle.com

Copyright © 2015 by Abby Eagle

Edition: 1/03/2015
put-insomnia-to-sleep.indd
put-insomnia-to-sleep-p.pdf

CreateSpace Assigned
ISBN-13:
978-1511919036

ISBN-10:
1511919035

Practise Meditation

Meditation has been shown to have a favourable influence on both serotonin and melatonin levels. Serotonin is associated with relaxation while melatonin regulates sleep.

Try and schedule in 10-30 minutes of meditation sometime in the evening and you will be greatly rewarded for it. Meditation does not just have to be about relaxation, it can also be used as a time to review the day and plan the next. You will find that it is far more effective to do this process sitting in meditation rather than lying in bed.

HOW TO PUT INSOMNIA TO SLEEP

And get a good nights sleep every night

CONTENTS

PREFACE

Some people drop into a deep sleep the moment their head hits the pillow while others have to work hard to get to sleep and then get back to sleep when they wake up in the night. Chronic insomnia can have a negative effect upon the health but looking on the bright side, and speaking from personal experience, light sleepers are more likely to experience astral travelling, out of body experiences, and other psychic phenomena.

Perhaps nature intended for some of us to be light sleepers? So rather than seeing insomnia as a problem you might like to treat it as an opportunity to explore your consciousness.

And by the way the procedures in this book came out of my personal experimentation - and they do work for me - and I trust they will for you too. Have a good nights sleep.

Abby Eagle

1

INTRODUCTION

There is no better way to improve your sleep than to cultivate the attitude of a loving parent with a small child. For example, when it is time for the child to go to bed the parent says, "You have had a great day. You have played with all your toys, you did 'this' and you did 'that' but now it is time to go to sleep. Tomorrow is another day but right now it is time to go to sleep. Get into bed and make yourself comfortable." They then repeat what they just said, "You have had a great day. You have played with all your toys, and you did 'this' and you did 'that'. Tomorrow is another day but right now it is time to go to sleep. Turn over, close your eyes and go to sleep now."

But when the parent gets into bed they lie awake thinking and worrying to all hours of the night. If only they took the attitude of a loving parent with themself they would be off to sleep in no time at all. In this book you will learn how to hold intelligent conversations with your unconscious such that you can get the good nights sleep that you so deserve.

Deal with underlying issues

There are two types of insomnia. The first is difficulty in getting to sleep, the second is waking up in the night and having difficulty getting back to sleep. As always, with any type of health problem it would be prudent to seek the opinion of a medical practitioner and rule out any underlying health issues. In addition you may need to address:

- Hot and humid weather.
- Eating too late in the evening.
- Poor diet and nutrient depletion.
- Exposure to mobile phone, television or computer screens before bed.
- LED lights on electrical equipment.
- Too much light in the bedroom. The bedroom is not dark enough.
- Street lights, car headlights, neighbours lights, moonlight.
- Feeling stressed and tense.
- Stimulants such as tea, green tea, coffee, chocolate, alcohol, cola and energy drinks.

There may be issues such as:

- Worry and anxiety.
- An overactive mind.
- A fear of dying in your sleep.
- A fear of being hurt while asleep.

- A fear of nightmares.
- A fear of something interfering with your sleep.
- Identifying with someone who had insomnia.
- Self punishment.
- Thoughts of a past negative event.
- Secondary gain. That is, the insomnia serves a purpose.
- A poor sleep strategy.

Be total in your sleeping

As the contemporary Zen mystic Osho has stated so many times, "Be total in whatever you do." When eating just eat, when drinking just drink, when walking just be the walking, when reading be totally involved in the reading, when dancing be total in the dance, if watching television then watch television - just learn to be totally present in whatever you do. The task is to be single pointed, to look neither left nor right, to put aside all distractions, to be so totally absorbed in an activity that you come into the present, into the here and now.

It may help to practise creating a boundary system for each and every activity, such that each and every activity has its own unique mental and physical state. That is, when eating keep your mind focussed on the process of eating. When eating avoid watching television, driving a vehicle or holding conversations that involve a lot of thinking. Each of those activities is a discrete state in itself. If you are having a social drink with your friends then avoid discussing work or serious topics. Schedule those topics of discussion to another time. Be clear when you begin and complete an activity so that you don't carry one state into another, as can happen in family situations where parents may find themselves multitasking various activities and blur work, home duties, parenting and relationships, such that the parents feel like they don't get any quality time for themselves. When preparing food, prepare the food. When eating the family meal then switch off the television and sit at a table. In this way you define each activity. When dinner is over then dinner is finished, then it is time to engage in another activity - even relaxation can be demarcated as an activity.

When reading a book learn to focus in on the book and keep your mind on what you are reading. If your mind wanders onto unrelated topics then bring it back to what you have in front of you. Don't be thinking about other things. In this way you learn to create a boundary system around each activity such that you can do your absolute best in that activity. Likewise, sleep is a time to forget the world and to get lost in the process of sleeping. As soon as you are ready for sleep then all thoughts should be conducive to sleep. There should be no thoughts of what happened that day or what might happen the next. In addition there should be no statements that presuppose a difficulty in getting to sleep, for example:

- I <u>need</u> to get to sleep.

- I <u>must</u> get to sleep.
- I <u>have</u> to get to sleep.
- I <u>can't</u> get to sleep.
- I <u>can't</u> relax.
- That 'noise' is keeping me awake.

Those types of thoughts will only serve to fuel the insomnia. Instead all of your thoughts should support your desired outcome, for example:

- I am going to focus all of my energy on getting to sleep.
- It's time to concentrate on getting to sleep.
- It's time to relax and go to sleep.
- It's time to get to sleep.
- I am going to have a good night's sleep.
- I am going to go straight to sleep and sleep soundly all through the night.

So learning how to get a good night's sleep is going to involve learning how to master your thought processes. If you are still awake after ten minutes then ask yourself, "Am I focussed on getting to sleep or am I thinking about other things?" If you have been thinking about other things then remind yourself that you need to bring your total attention to getting to sleep. You may need to do this over and over again until you learn to master your mind and master your state.

Make positive suggestions that lead towards sleep

To begin, I'd like you to say to yourself, "See yourself taking a deep breath." Do that right now. What happens? Did you find yourself taking a deep breath? If not, then repeat it a number of times until your unconscious mind accepts the suggestion and you find yourself taking a deep breath.

Now think the word, "Yawn", and see if your unconscious mind responds by having you yawn. Think the word, "Yawn", once again. Did you find yourself yawning again? What does this tell you? You think to yourself, "See yourself taking a deep breath", and you find yourself taking a deep breath. Then you think to yourself, "Yawn", and you find yourself yawning. Perhaps those people who sleep well are just better at suggesting to themselves to go to sleep. Perhaps they are just more experienced in using self hypnosis? Okay, now it's time to find which suggestions work the best for you.

Think to yourself, "Take a deep breath". How deep was the breath? Was it a shallow breath or a deep breath? Now think to yourself, "Yawn". Did you have a small or a large physiological response? What you want to do is discover which suggestions bring about the strongest response. Now think to yourself, "Relax". What was the response? Big or small? Now think to yourself, "Sleep". What was your response? Which suggestion got you the biggest response?

Now in turn repeat each of those suggestions about five to ten times. For example, "Take a deep breath... take a deep breath... take a deep breath... take a deep breath... take a deep breath." Give it a few seconds between each suggestion. Now repeat to yourself, "Yawn... yawn... yawn... yawn... yawn... yawn... yawn... yawn... yawn... yawn." "Sleep... sleep... sleep... sleep... sleep... sleep... sleep... sleep."

By now the understanding should be arising that your unconscious mind is always listening and has been responding to your self talk all of your life. If a word like 'yawn' can bring about a positive physiological response then it stands to reason that other words may have a negative response so bring awareness to your thought processes and choose carefully what you think about. Make a decision to have positive thoughts. Lift up your right hand and repeat after me, "From this day forth I want to think happy thoughts, loving thoughts, kind thoughts, playful thoughts, healthy thoughts and peaceful thoughts. I want to think thoughts that reward me, that esteem me, that value me, that make me feel good - thoughts that bring me a sense of happiness and well being.

If at times you find that your mind is particularly busy with unnecessary thoughts it may help to give suggestions to switch off the mind, to shut down the mind, to turn off the waking thought processes and to go to sleep. In my case when I do this, in my mind I see lights being switched off. For example, street lights being switched off, lights in a high rise property being switched off, lights in a house being switched off, and so forth. I also hear machines and motors being switched off, and I hear and feel the vibrations come to a standstill.

In some cases it may help to give yourself permission to go to sleep quickly even though you may not be perfectly comfortable and even though their may be distracting noises. Repeat to yourself over and over again: relaxing peacefully... resting peacefully... sleeping peacefully... dreaming peacefully...

2

SLEEP PROCEDURE 'A' TRANSCRIPT

(Long version)

Step 1. Before you get into bed

When it is time to go to bed say the following out aloud: "I am now going to bed. I am ready to go to sleep." When you get into your bedroom say, "In a moment I am going to get into bed. I am going to make myself comfortable then I will reflect upon the day's activities for a few minutes. I will feel satisfied that I did my best today and that I expect to have an even better day tomorrow. Then I will begin to relax. The relaxation will deepen and spread throughout my entire body. The same quality of relaxation will spread to my mind and my mind will become quiet. Then I will go to sleep and I will sleep soundly throughout the entire night, and I will awaken in the morning feeling refreshed and energised."

Support the dialogue with a visualisation. Make an image and get a sense of yourself going to sleep. See yourself sleeping peacefully throughout the night and waking at a specified time in the morning feeling happy that you slept well.

Step 2. On getting into bed watch the breath

Get into bed and make yourself comfortable. In your mind say the following to yourself: "I am now in bed and making myself comfortable. I learned a lot today. I achieved x, y and z. I am satisfied that I did my best. Tomorrow I will do even better."

Close your eyes and turn your attention to watching the breathing of your body. You will find it easiest if you watch the breathing in the region of the diaphragm and belly. To watch the breath you don't concentrate on it or change the breathing - all you do is notice the breathing of the body. This will work to slow the thoughts of the mind and when you realise that you have been distracted by your thoughts you bring your awareness back to the breathing. "Now I am going to watch the breathing in my body and I will keep on watching the breathing until I wake up in the morning."

Step 3. Eye closure

"As long as I watch the breathing in my body the muscles around my eyes will relax to the extent that I won't be able to open my eyes. As long as I watch the breathing I won't be able to open my eyes. I am now going to test my eyes to see if I can't open them." You know that you could open the eyes but that is not what you want. What you want is for the eyes to remain closed as long as you watch the breathing. When you try and open the eyes and you can not then you have achieved what is known as eye closure. At various stages of the sleep procedure you might like to test for other muscle groups. For example, to try and move an arm or a leg. When the muscles fail to respond to your conscious commands then you have what is known as catalepsy. Catalepsy is an indicator of trance and it is a part of going to sleep now.

Step 4. Relax the rest of the body

So you continue, "Now I am going to take the same quality of relaxation that I have around my eyes and spread that to the rest of my face. My face is now becoming totally relaxed. Totally relaxed. I am now going to double that relaxation. And double the relaxation once again." Remember to keep your awareness on the breathing.

"Now I am going to take that same quality of relaxation that I have around my eyes and face, and spread that to my neck and shoulders. My neck and shoulders are now becoming totally relaxed. Totally relaxed. I am now going to double that relaxation. And double the relaxation again.

"Now I am going to take that same quality of relaxation that I have around my eyes, face, neck and shoulders, and spread that to my right arm. My right arm is now becoming totally relaxed. Totally relaxed. I am now going to double that relaxation. And double the relaxation again. I know that I could move my right arm but that is not what I want to do. What I want is for the arm to be so totally relaxed that it won't work.

My arm is now totally relaxed." Remember to keep your awareness on the breathing.

"Now I am going to take that same quality of relaxation that I have around my eyes and spread that to my left arm. My left arm is now becoming totally relaxed. Totally relaxed. I am now going to double that relaxation. And double the relaxation again. I know that I could move my left arm but that is not what I want to do. What I want is for the arm to be so totally relaxed that it won't work. My arm is now totally relaxed.

"Now I am going to take that same quality of relaxation that I have around my eyes and spread that to my torso, chest, back and breathing. My torso, chest, back and breathing are now becoming totally relaxed. Totally relaxed. I am now going to double that relaxation, and double the relaxation again." Remember to keep your awareness on the breathing.

"Now I am going to take that same quality of relaxation that I have around my eyes and spread that to my legs and feet. My legs and feet are now becoming totally relaxed. Totally relaxed. I am now going to double that relaxation. And double the relaxation again."

Step 5. Banish the thoughts from the mind
"Now that I have relaxed my body it's time to spread this same quality of relaxation to my mind. What I am going to do is to banish the thoughts from my mind

so that it becomes as silent as the moment just before I go to sleep. I am now turning down the volume on the thoughts in my mind. My internal dialogue is becoming quieter and quieter. The voice is going further away and fading into the distance."

Repeat. "I am now turning down the volume on the thoughts in my mind. My internal dialogue is becoming quieter and quieter. The internal dialogue is going further away and fading into the distance." Keep on turning down the volume of the internal dialogue, make it go further away and fade off into the distance.

"I am now turning down the images in my mind. The pictures are becoming darker. They are fading and moving off into the distance." Repeat. "I am now turning down the images in my mind. The images are becoming darker. They are fading and moving off into the distance. I am banishing all of the thoughts from my mind. All of the thoughts are now disappearing from my mind. My mind is becoming absolutely silent – just like that moment I enter into just before I drift off to sleep." Remember to keep your awareness on the breathing at all times.

"As long as I keep my awareness on the breathing all of the thoughts will disappear from my mind." Repeat. "As long as I keep my awareness on the breathing all of the thoughts will disappear from my mind and I will enter into that space of silence just like before I go to sleep."

Step 6. Relax down the levels

"Now, even though my mind and body are becoming very relaxed I know that I can relax even further. If relaxation had a number of levels then let's say that right now I am at level one. What I want to do is to relax right down to the deepest depths of relaxation. As I float down a level the relaxation will double.

"I am now at level one of relaxation and I am now floating down to level two. The relaxation is doubling. I am now doubling the relaxation. I am now at the second level of relaxation.

"But I know that I can relax even more so I am going to float down to the next level and double the relaxation once again. I am now floating down to the third level and the relaxation is doubling. I am now at the third level of relaxation and my mind is becoming very quiet.

"I know that I can relax even more so I am going to double this relaxation once again. I am now floating down to the fourth level of relaxation and as I do so the relaxation will double and my mind will become even more quiet. I am now doubling the relaxation. I am now at the fourth level of relaxation.

"But I know that there are deeper levels of relaxation than this. Each time I float down a level the relaxation will automatically double and my mind will become even more quiet. All I have to do is say the number of the next level and my unconscious mind will deepen the relaxation even more and I will enter deeper into that space of silence that I enter into just before I drift off to sleep."

Float down the levels just by saying the number and notice how the relaxation deepens with each level. Do this at your own speed. 'Five, six, seven…'" Notice how all you have to do is keep your awareness on the breath and say the next number, and your unconscious mind will automatically take you deeper.

Step 7. Suggestion to go to sleep

"Okay, now that my mind and body are totally relaxed it is time for me to go to sleep. I can feel myself drifting off to sleep. And I know that as long as I keep my awareness on the breathing nothing will bother me and I will sleep soundly throughout the night and awake in the morning feeling refreshed and energised."

3

WHAT TO DO IF YOU HAVE A HABIT OF WAKING UP IN THE NIGHT?

You can be woken up for a number of reasons. Snoring and sleep apnea - which may be related to food allergies, a need to visit the toilet, physical discomfort, being too hot or cold, wind, rain, noises and so on. Putting these types of reasons aside for the moment, if you find yourself waking up for no apparent reason then self hypnosis may help.

When you are ready to go to sleep then address your unconscious mind. Give suggestions to sleep through the entire night and not to be woken by a dream or a fear. Sometimes the unconscious may try and protect you from a bad dream by having you wake up. If this is the case then suggest to the unconscious mind that you want it to dream the dream and to process it and to allow you to continue your restful sleep.

If the habit is to wake at 2:30am then give the suggestion to sleep a bit longer and not to wake until perhaps 4:00 - 4:30am. Once you have achieved that then give the suggestion to not to wake until 5:00 - 5:30am, and so on. So that each night the sleep pattern gradually improves. When you communicate with your unconscious mind you should be alert for ideomotor responses. (See the glossary for an explanation.)

Then give suggestions to, "See yourself drifting off to sleep. See yourself sleeping all the way through the night. Unconscious mind sometimes you wake me at 2:30am. What I want you to do now is to keep me fast asleep until 3:00 - 3:30am. If in the past you have been protecting me from a bad dream then what I want you to do now is to keep me fast asleep and to process that dream. Do you understand?"

In some cases you may wake up on cue to a noise or sound. For example, a mother can be fast asleep yet wake up at the sound of her baby crying in another room. This indicates that the unconscious mind never really goes to sleep, only the conscious mind and body do so. It is well known that under anaesthetic a patient is able to hear everything that medical staff say, and recall this information under hypnosis at a later date. In some cases, such as in a near death experience, the patient may also have a visual representation of what happened. When knocked unconscious a person is able to hear everything that is going on around them and they may be able to recall this information under hypnosis depending upon the severity of the injury.

However, in the normal course of things you may not want to have your sleep disturbed by wind, rain, a creaking roof, a flyscreen door banging in the wind, neighbours coming home late or leaving for work early, the sound of a neighbours gate, a garbage truck, a refrigerator and so forth. These are environmental sounds that you have no control over but which pose no threat to your wellbeing. In which case it may be useful to preframe all likely disturbances and suggest to your unconscious mind that when you hear these sounds that you will remain asleep. You should also add the suggestions that if you do need to wake up for an emergency that you will do so easily. You may need to list each sound and make a specific suggestion to the unconscious mind that it is okay to go to sleep while those sounds are there and in addition to remain asleep, so that they do not disturb your rest. You should specify which sounds should be ignored and which sounds should wake you up. You may need to train your unconscious mind over a period of time. When a noise disturbs you then say to yourself, "It is safe. It is okay. This noise is not going to bother me at all. When I hear this noise I want my unconscious mind to keep me fast asleep. Go to sleep now." Repeat this type of suggestion to yourself every time a noise disturbs you.

◊ Case notes: Being conscious of the external world while asleep (28/06/2011)

"It is about 7:30am. I can hear someone out on the street. Someone comes through the front gate. I recognise the sounds of the lawn mower contractors. There are footsteps, the sounds of a mower being wheeled along the path, and then the mower starts up. A few minutes later my alarm goes off and I wake up, and then I realise that in fact I had been fast asleep - yet I had been fully conscious of the activity outside my bedroom window."

◊ Case notes: Giving suggestions to remain asleep while asleep (30/06/2011)

"I am aware that I am asleep and that I am stretching my legs in the bed and rolling from side to side. I can feel the bed clothes against my body and I am aware of my hands rearranging the bedclothes as I roll over. I am aware that it must be early morning because there is light on my eyelids and I can hear familiar noises outside. I don't want to wake up; I want to go deeper asleep so I say to myself, "Go deeper and deeper, deeper and deeper." This experience is different to others that I had some years ago where I witnessed the body moving of its own accord; here I am actually consciously moving the body while asleep.

There is a period of dreaming. In one dream there is a landscape in front with an ocean in the background which extends all the way to the horizon. My perspective on it is from a higher angle than normal, something like an artist might paint, it is like the ocean is too high in the sky. A friend, Vince, is in a dark building. I call out to him to come and watch a surfer who has taken off at a point break to the left and is rapidly surfing miles across the horizon to the right. I am explaining to Vince that what we are seeing is not real because in reality the surfer would not move so fast across the horizon. There is some sort of parallax error. Then the alarm clock goes off and I wake up.

The ocean usually symbolises for me the ocean of consciousness. In this dream it is like the surfer is surfing the ocean of consciousness. Vince comes out of the darkness into the light. There is also an awareness that the dreamscape is not real."

Read more at www.abbyeagle.com/blog/

4

SLEEP PROCEDURE 'B' TRANSCRIPT

(Short version)

Step 1. Familiarise yourself with the long procedure

Once you are familiar with the longer relaxation procedure then you can use this shorter procedure. Start by getting into bed and affirming that you are ready to sleep.

Step 2. Eye closure

Close your eyes and watch the breathing. Get eye closure and hold onto the relaxation. This induces a trance state. Then deepen the trance state with a breathing technique as follows:

Step 3. Deep breathing

Keep your awareness on the breathing. Take a deep breath and hold it for the count of ten. You might feel sensations of warmth in your body. This an indicator of cellular respiration. As you breath out send a wave of relaxation all the way to your toes. Breath normally for about three breaths then take another deep breath. Hold it for the count of ten then relax, and as you breath out send a wave of relaxation all the way through your body, down to your toes, doubling the relaxation as you do so.

Repeat the above procedure about ten or so times.

Step 4. Check eye closure

Now check for eye closure. You should have perfect eye closure. If not, then watch the breathing in the body and notice that as long as you watch the breathing in the body that you can not open your eyes.

Step 5. Banish the thoughts from the mind

The next step is to banish the thoughts from the mind. Suggest to your self that as long as you watch the breathing all of the thoughts will disappear from the mind. 'As long as I watch my breathing all the thoughts will disappear and fade from my mind. All the thoughts are now fading from my mind and my mind is becoming very quiet.' Turn down the volume on the internal dialogue. Put the internal dialogue way off into the distance and let it fade from your mind. Darken the pictures in your mind then turn them down so that they become very small and then let them fade off into the distance. Repeat this process a number of times with the last suggestion being that even the part of you that is giving the suggestions will also be quiet. With practise, by holding the feeling you can give a suggestion that you would normally have done with words. "All the thoughts are now fading from my mind and my mind is becoming very quiet. Unconscious mind banish all the thoughts from my mind so that my mind becomes absolutely quiet. Let me enter that space of silence that I enter into just before going to sleep."

Step 6. Suggest that you will drift off to sleep

Keep watching the breath at all times. Suggest to yourself that as long as you watch the breathing that the silence in your mind, and the relaxation in your body will take you deep into that space of silence that you experience just before going to sleep. Say to yourself, "See yourself drifting off to sleep now."

Step 7. Float down levels of relaxation

The next step is to float down through levels of relaxation. The level that you start at is level one. You then progressively float down through levels of relaxation. As you float down a level the relaxation in your body doubles and the silence in your mind deepens. At first you make suggestions to yourself that as you float down to the next level that the relaxation will double but once you have counted down to level five, or even earlier, all you need do is to say the next number and then feel the relaxation deepening. This procedure will take you into a very deep state. Both body and mind will become very quiet.

Step 8. Suggest that you will drift off to sleep

Once you have floated down enough levels, and while watching the breathing suggest to yourself that it is time to go to sleep. "As long as I watch my breathing I will find myself drifting off to sleep. I will sleep the deepest that I have ever slept and I will sleep all the way through the night. In the morning I will awaken feeling refreshed, alert and energised." In addition add, "See yourself drifting off to sleep now."

Step 9. Reinforce your success and go back to sleep

If you wake up in the night congratulate yourself on having relaxed yourself to sleep. Then do a short summary of the relaxation procedure: start by watching the breath, check eye closure, take a few deep breaths to deepen the state, banish the thoughts from your mind, float down a number of levels to become even deeper relaxed then suggest to yourself, 'See yourself drifting off to sleep."

5

SLEEP PROCEDURE 'C' - MOVE AWARENESS TO THE FEET

An overactive mind indicates in one sense that you are out of touch with the body. In this extension of the previous sleep procedures you learn to shift your awareness from the mind to the feet. Once you master this procedure you should find yourself drifting off to sleep within a few minutes, and getting back to sleep quickly if you should wake up again in the night. However, it can not be repeated enough that if you want to master your mind then you have to bring awareness to your internal processes. Which means, that as soon as you are aware that you are not asleep then run the procedure, for if you remain lost in the mind then nothing will work.

Procedure
1. Relax the muscles around the eyes.
2. Spread relaxation down through the body.
3. Relax the thoughts from the mind. Turn down the internal dialogue, etc.
4. Give suggestion to, "Go to sleep now."
5. Repeat steps 1-3 and add, "Relaxing all the way

down to the tips of my toes. "

Note that in this procedure rather than saying, "Relax my eyes", you say, "Relax the eyes." Say it as if you were addressing another person.

Get into bed, make yourself comfortable, set an intention to go to sleep and then repeat the following script softly and rapidly in your mind: "It is time to go to sleep now. Close your eyes and relax the muscles around the eyes... keep on relaxing the muscles around the eyes... keep on relaxing the muscles around the eyes... keep on relaxing the muscles around the eyes... keep on relaxing the muscles around the eyes... keep on relaxing the muscles around the eyes... keep on relaxing the muscles around the eyes until the eyes will no longer work..."

Test to see whether you have eye closure and then continue:

"Now go to sleep... go to sleep... and relax the muscles around the eyes... keep on relaxing the muscles around the eyes... and take that quality of relaxation and spread it all the way down the body to the tips of your fingers and the tips of your toes...

"Keep on relaxing the muscles around the eyes... keep on relaxing the muscles around the eyes... keep on relaxing the muscles around the eyes... and take that quality of relaxation and spread it all the way down the body to the tips of your fingers and the tips of your toes...

"Keep on relaxing the muscles around the eyes... keep on relaxing the muscles around the eyes... keep on relaxing the muscles around the eyes... and take that quality of relaxation and put it into the mind and relax all the thoughts from the mind... turning down the internal dialogue... letting it get quieter and quieter... quieter and quieter... quieter and quieter... slowing down the internal dialogue... letting it get slower and slower... slower and slower... slower and slower... soften the internal dialogue... letting it get softer and softer... let it become more warm, more loving, more friendly... keep on turning down the internal dialogue... let it become very small... let it become very tiny... relaxing all thoughts from the mind and entering into that space of silence you enter into just before you drift off to sleep now...

"Keep on relaxing the muscles around the eyes... keep on relaxing the muscles around the eyes and spread that quality of relaxation all the way down to the tips of your fingers and the tips of your toes..."

Imagine that you have one foot in a bucket of cold water and ice. Wiggle your toes in the bucket of water. Feel the ice blocks and the sensation of coldness. Imagine that your other foot is in a bucket of hot water. Wiggle your foot in the hot water and feel the warmth penetrating deep into the foot. After one minute switch each feet to the other bucket. Alternate from cold to hot a few times then finish with both feet in a bucket of hot water. Feel the warmth rising up your legs. Tell yourself that it is time to go to sleep.

From the mind to the body

1. The rationale of the hot and cold water treatment is that the concentration required to imagine and sense a difference in temperature in a part of the body withdraws the energy from the mind, hence quietening it. In another respect the energy is moved from the mind to the heart.

2. There is a natural therapies procedure in which one sits in a small bath (a sitz bath) just big enough so that the water reaches to the navel and half way up the thighs. In one procedure, one sits in a bath of hot water with the feet in a bath of cold water. After 15-60 seconds you change position and sit in the cold water and put your feet in the hot water. This procedure of alternating hot and cold baths may be repeated about five or six times. We utilise that principle in the following procedure.

3. The following section gives you some additional procedures that you can add onto the end of the deep trance procedure, or use in place of the deep trance procedure.

Alternating hands and feet

Imagine that you put your left finger tips into cold water. Slowly insert your hand deeper into the water all the way up to the elbow. Then imagine that you put your right toes into cold water and slowly immerse your leg up to the knee. Then imagine that you put your right finger tips into hot water and then the arm all the way to the elbow. Imagine that you put your left toes into hot water and immerse the leg all the way up to the knee. So your left hand and right foot are in cold water, and your right hand and left foot are in hot water. Run this procedure in your mind for a few minutes to reinforce the experience then alternate from hot to cold, and from cold to hot. Periodically suggest to yourself that it is time to go to sleep.

Then imagine that you put the left leg and arm into hot water, and the right leg and arm into cold water. After a while reverse the procedure so that the left leg and arm go into cold water and the right arm and leg go into hot water.

To finish, imagine stepping both feet into hot water all the way up to the waist, and putting both hands into cold water. After a period of time alternate.

If you have a kidney problem then it might not be such a good idea to imagine that your feet are in cold water. Instead visualise a source of heat on the soles of your feet. For example, an electric bar heater or a wood fuelled fire. Imagine that the heater is close to the soles of both feet. Feel your feet becoming quite hot. For a contrast imagine that your hands are dipped in cold water.

If hot weather is making it difficult to get to sleep then it may help to imagine that you are somewhere very cold, such as a walk-in freezer, or lying on a bed of snow, or dipping your hands into an esky of ice and ice cold water, or some such contrasting experience. Likewise if you happen to find yourself in the situation where you are cold it can help to imagine that you are somewhere very hot.

Wash your feet

Imagine that you shower one foot up to the calf using a warm hand held shower then wash the foot thoroughly with a soapy flannel. Shower the soap off and then wash the foot once again with the soapy flannel. Dry the foot with a nice soft towel making sure that you work between the toes. Repeat with the other foot. Then suggest to yourself that it is time to go to sleep.

Massage your feet

Imagine that someone is massaging your feet. Then suggest to your self that you go to sleep.

Drop down into the heart

Get a sense that you can drop down from the mind into the heart and then into 'being' in the belly.

Hear music playing in your toes

Imagine music is playing in your toes and feet. Rather than trying to hear the music playing in the location of your feet try and get the sense that you can feel the vibration of the music, the energy of the music playing in the feet. Invite the music to slowly play up through the body.

Then reach up into the universal source of love and healing energy, seeing and feeling the love and healing energy to be pouring down through your crown chakra as a golden liquid into your heart, filling your heart with the love and healing energy until your heart radiates a brilliant golden light, and see and feel the love and healing energy flowing all the way through your body to the tips of your fingers and the tips of your toes.

Repeat the procedure. Reaching up into the source of universal love and healing energy, as if you are under a massive water fall, and see and feel the love and healing energy to be showering down over you, saturating your entire body and clothing with the love and healing energy, until your entire body and clothing radiate a brilliant golden light.

Feel the music playing up inside the body from the tips of your toes while the love and healing energy pours down over you from above. Then suggest to your self that you go to sleep.

Find a bed buddy
Some people find that a *bed buddy pillow* gives them something soft to cuddle up to. Alternatively you might try a pillow under your legs, feet, knees or between your knees.

Relax the muscles in the feet
The long sleep procedure *(Sleep procedure 'A' transcript)* begins with relaxing the muscles around the eyes and then progressively spreading that quality of relaxation down through the body to the feet.

As an option you may like to start by relaxing the muscles in the feet and toes until the toes are totally relaxed. When the toes are totally relaxed then progressively spread that relaxation up through the ankles, legs and torso to the eyelids.

Turn down the mind
In this procedure you bring your awareness to the internal dialogue until it disappears, enter into the silence and then go to sleep. Begin with, "I have had a good day, now it is time to go to sleep". Then turn down the internal dialogue until it disappears or at least until it becomes quieter. Then bring your awareness to the internal dialogue until it stops. Maintain the no-mind state and remain with the silence. Step into the silence and drop deeper into the silence. Then give a suggestion to go to sleep.

The Mind Director Procedure

Imagine that you have a control panel at your finger tips, much like a graphic equaliser. There are slider controls and dials for the tempo, tonality and volume. You need to move your fingers and your hand in the much the same way that you would do this in reality.

Start by tuning into some negative internal dialogue. Imagine that you have an imaginary control panel at your finger tips - turn the volume down. Let it get quieter and quieter, quieter and quieter. Slow down the tempo. Let it get slower and slower, slower and slower. Soften the tonality. Let it get softer and softer, softer and softer. Let the internal dialogue become more friendly and loving.

Turn down the volume. Let it get quieter and quieter, quieter and quieter. Slow down the tempo. Let it get slower and slower, slower and slower. Soften the tonality. Let it become more friendly and loving. Let it get softer and softer. Turn the volume all the way down. Let it become very small. Put the internal dialogue all the way out on the horizon. Banishing all thoughts from the mind and entering into that space of silence that you enter into just before you drift off to sleep.

And now just turn up the silence. Let the silence become a little bigger, a little deeper, and a little more profound. Remain with the silence, and enjoy the feelings of peace and relaxation that come with a silent no mind - and then say, "Go to sleep now".

Once you are familiar with using an imaginary control panel to manage the self talk, that is to turn down, slow down, soften and move the internal dialogue out to the horizon, then all you need do is move your hand to indicate that you are doing just that. So, one does not need to say anything in the mind - one just sets the intention to turn down, slow down, soften and move the internal dialogue out into the distance, and then you just move your hand to indicate that you are doing just that. This is enough in itself to suggest to the unconscious mind what you want it to do. In this way you will find that it only takes a few minutes for the mind to quieten and for you to enter a no-mind state. As the silence deepens then give suggestions to yourself to turn down the mind and to slow down the mind. As you do so you should notice that you go deeper and deeper. If you have set the intention to go to sleep then sleep should follow within a few minutes. If you plan to use this procedure for meditation then you will find yourself entering into deep meditation.

◊ Case notes: How to gain control of a racing mind

"Sometimes you may need to work with your current experience before doing a relaxation technique. For example, one night I was having difficulty getting to sleep and when I tried self hypnosis I had difficulty getting eye closure so I worked with my current experience.

My mind was in high gear (a trance state in itself) so I deepened this state by suggesting to myself that my mind was like a racing train. As I made these suggestions to myself an image formed from the film *Train*. Two men were fighting on the top of the train trying to gain control of it. They tried to block my path to the engine but I bypassed them and went straight to the engine compartment. My view was from the outside. The engine compartment was glassed up and there was no driver. An image of the bad terminator from the *Terminator 2* film came to mind. He punched a hole in the window, turned his body to liquid and flowed through the hole into the compartment. He tried to stop the train but the controls failed to respond. So I went to the engine compartment and threw water on the fire (it was a steam engine). As the fire went out the train slowed. My mind also slowed down and I was able to get to sleep.

This process worked by using hypnosis to pace the current experience in order to gain control over it and then lead to my desired outcome. When I thought of my racing mind it only seemed natural to draw the analogy of a racing train. If you have a problem with a racing mind use what ever analogy fits for you.

6

SLEEP PROCEDURE 'D' - REINDUCE A DRUG STATE

Your body remembers every drug that you have taken. Whether that be alcohol, a recreational drug, an anaesthetic or a sleeping pill. This can be particularly useful when you want the effect of the drug but not the side effects. This sleep procedure works by having you reaccess the experience of having taken a sleeping pill or a muscle relaxant, and tracking the sequence of body sensations that lead to sleep.

Procedure
Step 1. Think of a drug. As you think of having taken that drug remember what you could see, hear and feel at the time.

Step 2. If the drug came in a bubble pack then see, hear and feel the pill/tablet being popped out of the pack. If the drug came in a bottle, see, hear and feel the unscrewing of the lid, and the sound of the pills as you tip one into your hand.

Step 3. Remember the experience of putting the pill/tablet into your mouth. Does it have a taste? Remember the taste. Do you chew or suck the pill/

tablet? Do you wash it down with liquid? Go through the exact sequence of remembering the experience as vividly as you can in pictures, sounds, feelings, smells and taste. The following steps are very important.

Step 4. What is the first sensation in your body that lets you know that you have taken that drug and you are on your way to sleep? Where is that sensation located in the body? Feel that sensation as vividly as you can.

Step 5. What is the next sensation and where is that located?

Step 6. Keep on following the sequence of sensations and their location. There will be at the most only four or five locations. Track them all. The last sensation should be that of drifting off to sleep.

Step 7. Rerun the entire procedure a number of times, taking time to fully experience each step.

Step 8. Anchor the beginning of the strategy with the name of the drug followed by the word 'sleep'. Thereafter whenever you say the name of the drug and follow it with the word 'sleep' you should find yourself naturally relaxing towards a state of sleep.

7

DEEP SLEEP MEDITATION TRANSCRIPT

If you have a problem with being a light sleeper and of waking up in the night then the following script should help you to drop into deeper levels of sleep. At the least it should help you to improve your self hypnosis and meditation skills, as the upside of being a light sleeper is that it gives you an opportunity to practise your meditation skills even while asleep, something which a deep sleeper probably never even *dreamed* of.

In the last paragraph of the *Deep Sleep Meditation Transcript* there is a statement, "You are now fast asleep." It might seem like a strange statement to make but the witnessing consciousness never goes to sleep. The witnessing consciousness is always awake. What nature intends by sleep is for the physical body to rest and restore itself; and for the mind to quieten down. The one who is aware of the body being awake is the same as the one who is aware of the dreaming. In fact, on occasions you may be aware that you are asleep and dreaming. So the statement, "You are now fast asleep.", is intended to convey that it is the witnessing consciousness that is learning how to drive the mind and body.

You should aim to memorise the following script. As with the other scripts in this manual, some parts could be said slowly while other parts could be said rapidly, but no matter the speed, speak to yourself softy and gently.

Transcript

"Close your eyes... and relax the muscles around the eyes until the eyes will no longer work... keep on relaxing the muscles around the eyes... keep on relaxing the muscles around the eyes... keep on relaxing the muscles around the eyes... keep on relaxing the muscles around the eyes until the eyes will no longer work... when you are sure that the eyes will no longer work what I want you to do is to try and open the eyes and discover you cannot... close the eyes and keep on relaxing the muscles around the eyes... keep on relaxing the muscles around the eyes... keep on relaxing the muscles around the eyes... now take the quality of relaxation that you have around the eyes and spread it to your cheeks, your lips, your teeth, your jaw and head, neck and shoulders... keep on relaxing the muscles around the eyes... and take the quality of relaxation that you have around your eyes and spread it all the way down through the body to the tips of your fingers and the tips of your toes...

"Keep on relaxing the muscles around the eyes...

keep on relaxing the muscles around the eyes... and now turn down the internal dialogue... don't think about turning down the internal dialogue, just turn it down... letting it get quieter and quieter... quieter and quieter... quieter... turn down the internal dialogue... letting it get smaller and smaller... smaller and smaller... smaller and smaller... slow down the internal dialogue... slow it right down and when the internal dialogue slows right down you might find a yawn coming to your throat... keep on turning down the volume... slow it down... soften the internal dialogue... let it get softer and softer... softer and softer... softer and softer... let the internal dialogue sort of flatten out... let it become more friendly and loving... turn the internal dialogue all the way down until it totally disappears... put the internal dialogue all the way out on the horizon... banishing all thoughts from the mind and entering into that space of silence that you enter into just before you drift off to sleep...

"Keep on relaxing the muscles around the eyes... keep on relaxing the muscles around the eyes... and take this quality of relaxation that you have around the eyes and put it into the mind and relax all the thoughts from the mind... just relaxing all the thoughts from the mind... allowing this coaching internal dialogue to become very small... to relax and totally disappear now... entering into that space of silence that you enter into just before you drift off to sleep now...

"Relaxing all tension from the body... turning down

the internal dialogue... turning down the tension in the body... letting the tension get smaller and smaller... smaller and smaller... relaxing... fading... putting the tension all the way out on the horizon... relaxing the tension from the body... feeling the tension gradually weaken and get softer and softer... feeling the tension get smaller and smaller... feeling the tension continue to relax even more as it moves further out towards the horizon... the tension getting smaller and smaller as it disappears over the horizon... and dropping down under the tension... relaxing deeper and deeper... dropping down under the tension and entering into that space of silence that you enter into just before you drift off to sleep now...

"Relaxing deeper and deeper... deeper and deeper... deeper and deeper... drifting... floating... dreaming... dropping down deeper and deeper... dropping down into dream sleep... deeper and deeper into dream sleep... and now dropping down under the dream sleep... deeper and deeper... deeper and deeper... deeper and deeper... and continuing to drop down into deeper levels of sleep, deeper and deeper... and even deeper still now... into the deepest level of sleep and continuing to drop down even further... leaving all thoughts behind and entering into a space of profound silence... floating... drifting... deeper and deeper still into the depths of the silence...

"And when I float back up into dream sleep during the night can the unconscious mind have me drop down under the dreaming once again into even deeper levels of sleep... and continue to have me drop down under that level into even deeper levels of sleep... and continue to have me drop down, deeper and deeper... deeper and deeper now...

"You are now fast asleep... carry on sleeping... going deeper and deeper... deeper and deeper... you are now fast asleep... you can hear me but you can't wake up... listen carefully... if you should wake up in the night then immediately remind yourself to relax the muscles around the eyes... to turn down the internal dialogue... put the thinking all the way out on the horizon... and enter into that space of silence that you enter into just before you drift off to sleep... and then to continue dropping down deeper and deeper... deeper and deeper... now go to sleep..."

8

BUILD A POSITIVE COACHING INTERNAL DIALOGUE

You are not the mind, body or the emotions, you are the witnessing consciousness – that is you are the one who is aware of the mind, body and emotions. You, that is consciousness needs to become the master of the mind. The mind needs to be the servant. Another way of saying that is that we need to learn how to move from the back seat into the drivers seat of our lives.

There are many things in life that we have no control over but we can learn to control how we respond. This comes by practising mindfulness - by being more consciousness in everything that we do. We start by building in a positive coaching internal dialogue that supports you in achieving your desired outcomes.

We start with the sentence stem, "See yourself taking a deep breath." Notice how the breathing changes. Then think the word, "Yawn". Do you find yourself yawning? Repeat the word, 'yawn' in your mind a few times. You should find yourself yawning. What do you learn from this? The unconscious mind is always listening to and acting upon the conversations that you hold in your mind. So choose your thoughts carefully. Practise making suggestions throughout the day with single words and short phrases. Start with the suggestion to yawn. As the body responds and you find yourself yawning this becomes a ratifier that the unconscious mind is listening to and acting upon every thought that you have. Then say to yourself words like, relax, be at peace, feel loved, feel good now, concentrate, listen in. Say to yourself, "See yourself feeling confident, being loving, feeling happy, striding with confidence into the future, feeling wonderful, completing your projects, bringing people into your life, etc.

Show me the posture

Say to yourself, "Show me the posture of sleep, show me the muscle tension of sleep, show me the muscle relaxation of sleep, show me the physiology of sleep, show me the breath of sleep, show me the face of sleep. On a scale of zero to ten how strong is this state of relaxation right now? Good, now I want my unconscious mind to deepen the relaxation, have the relaxation expand a little, become even more profound. Once again show me the posture of a deep relaxing sleep, the posture of a relaxed meditative mind. Relaxing into deep sleep now, show me the posture of silence, the posture of calmness, of relaxation and of happiness.

The same language patterns can be used at throughout the day using the following sentence stems. Show me the posture of... show me the breathing of... show me the physiology of... show me the face of... For example, show me the breath of love, of gratitude, of peacefulness, of happiness, of confidence, of health, of financial freedom, of success, of joy and of boundless energy. Make direct suggestions to the unconscious mind, and notice how the body responds, especially the face and the breath.

Think of some happy memories then say to self, "See yourself moving through the coming days and weeks smiling and laughing. See yourself moving through the day with a growing sense of confidence in your self."

Find two end states that have meaning for you and stack them. For example, professional prestige and financial freedom. Now show me the physiology of professional prestige and financial freedom. Having professional prestige and financial freedom now how do you look at the world differently, what do you see, hear and feel now? Looking through the eyes of professional prestige and financial freedom how does the world look to you?

Put your thoughts out on the horizon

While going to sleep put your thoughts out on the horizon. One way to do this is to think of a time when you saw a couple of people talking in the distance but they were too far away for you to hear what they were saying.

Now take your own internal dialogue and put it in the same location as the people in the distance. There is no need to see yourself in the same location as the people. All you need do is imagine that your internal dialogue is off in the distance. As you do so you should find that it either becomes quieter or disappears totally. Once it disappears just remain with the silence. You know that you have been successful when you wake up in the morning and there is no habitual thinking. You can still think but it arises out of a conscious desire to think not from an out of control mechanism, like a radio running in the background.

Enter into sleep through dreaming

Another way to get to sleep is to shift your consciousness into the dream experience. Say to yourself, "Go to sleep now and enter into that space of silence that you enter into just before drifting off to sleep. Enter into dreaming, start dreaming, drifting, floating, dreaming".

On going to bed try and remember a dream from the night before. Say to yourself, "Time to start dreaming again." If you should wake up in the night then bring your mind back to what you were dreaming about and continue the dream. "Go to back to sleep now."

This procedure works by shifting your consciousness

from the waking conscious state into the unconscious mind. As you move into the dreaming of the unconscious mind the body goes to sleep. Notice the distinction though, that it does not imply that you go unconscious. You enter into sleep consciously, you enter into sleep with awareness.

Simplified sleep procedure

Tell yourself, "Time to go to sleep." Notice if you yawn or not in response to the suggestion then repeat to yourself three times, "Go to sleep." Repeat this procedure at intervals of two minutes. As you begin to drift off repeat to yourself, "Going deeper and deeper, deeper into sleep now." Then stop the self talk and maintain the silence by using the witnessing procedure as follows. Set an intention to silence the internal dialogue and maintain the silence for ten minutes. Then witness the internal dialogue so that it disappears. Bring your awareness to the silence and maintain it. After a few minutes of silence say once to self, "Go to sleep now." See the chapter titled, "Meditation Basics" for more information on how to silence the mind.

Let nature be your teacher

You might have noticed at one time that you were lying in bed thinking and then it began to rain or the wind began to blow through the trees an then you felt your consciousness shift, your mind quieted down and you thought to yourself, "I can get to sleep now."

- and you did. The exercises in this book are a means for you to do that process with awareness. To shift your awareness away from the internal dialogue to the silence and to enter into the silence.

Ask questions that demonstrate respect, responsibility and understanding

If thinking continues then question the thinking, as if you were questioning someone who talked over you in a conversation. What does the continued thinking demonstrate? Perhaps a lack of respect? Find a value to get leverage on yourself. Do you want to demonstrate respect to yourself? Can you just be quiet for a few minutes and lie there in silence?

Rather then using direct suggestions to relax, quieten the mind and go to sleep we now learn how to communicate with our unconscious mind by asking questions that invite the unconscious mind to run a process at the level of the unconscious mind. We are not creating a division in the mind by having a discussion with ourselves, an argument. Not two parts - not fighting with ourselves but holding the intention to achieve a predetermined outcome. As with the Mind Director control panel, we work in a singular fashion and ask questions of ourselves. We may or may not get a response from the unconscious mind that we understand. Using a generalisation, a response from the left brain would be in the form of language while a response from the right brain may be in the form of an image, a gut feeling or a knowing.

If the language centre is over active then getting involved in a discussion with ourselves may only serve to keep it over active. The procedures in this book are designed to help quieten the language centre in the left hemisphere and shift your energy more over to the right hemisphere.

What we need to do is to quieten down the rampant, habitual thoughts and build in a more conscious coaching internal dialogue that supports your mind, body and heart. So as when directing a question to another person – who may remain quiet as they process the question and may not reply with words but more with a look or a gesture – here we direct a question to the unconscious mind but we are not expecting any specific type of reply – specifically we are not expecting more internal dialogue. We need to become more receptive to listening to our inner silence – of listening to our feelings, our intuition, our knowing, our unconscious mind and our heart.

So we ask a question and just give some time for the unconscious mind to process the question. Then we ask another question. The outcome should be that the mind becomes silent and remains silent such that you then find that you drift off to sleep. This type of questioning technique can be used to deal with rampant internal dialogue, negative thinking, critical thinking, judgemental thinking, any thinking that is not serving you – for the purpose of bringing you more into the present moment such that you can concentrate your energies in the present moment and apply yourself 100% to the task at hand. Whether that be getting to sleep, answering email, making a phone call, holding a conversation with another person, addressing a boardroom meeting, giving a talk, performing on stage, playing sport, relaxing or making love.

What type of leader are you?
In a conversation with another person is your mind quiet or are you thinking about what to say next and constantly interrupting? Learn to be quiet when you listen to another person, that is quiet on the inside as well as not interrupting. Give yourself some tasks to do. Just listening without interrupting. Let the other person finish what they are saying. Rather than holding onto a question or answer in your mind, perhaps jot it down on paper, or just let the thought go. Just see what happens.

When going to sleep, is your mind busy? If you tell yourself to go to sleep does the rampant thinking continue? If you were to hold a conversation with a group of people would you demonstrate that you are listening by acknowledging and supporting or would you be inside your mind judging, planning a response and looking for an opportunity to interrupt and say what you want to say?

What type of team leader are you? Are you controlling? D you tell people what to do or do you welcome input? Do you have what it takes to allow others to express themselves? Can you put others before your self? Can you lead silently? Can you let go your thoughts and lead yourself silently towards sleep?

Do these thoughts serve me?

So if you are laying in bed ready to go to sleep but find yourself thinking about things then step one is to bring in awareness that you are thinking. Step two is to ask, "Is this thinking useful? Is this thinking serving me right now? Is this something that I have thought about before? Is this something that I need to resolve? Is this something that I could just forget about? Is this something that would be best dealt with at another time? Should I make a decision to deal with this at some better time? When would be the best time to deal with it? Can I put that thinking to rest right now? Should I be awake or asleep?" So you ask intelligent question that serve you.

If the thinking continues then ask, "Is this thinking a good use of my time right now? What should I be doing right now? What is going to be the consequences of thinking like this right now? Is that what I want? Why do I want to go to sleep? Why do I need to go to sleep? What are the benefits of a good nights sleep?"

We could ask the question, "Can the mind become

silent?" But this direct question can only get a yes or no response - and you may get a 'yes but' response. By carefully asking questions that invite the unconscious mind to access and mobilise internal resources new understandings will arise and out of these understandings you will naturally find yourself achieving the desired outcome – a quiet peaceful state of mind.

So we ask, "Do these thoughts serve me right now? If not then what thoughts would serve me? What are the thoughts that I need to hold in mind such that I find myself drifting off to sleep? What is the one thought that if it should arise in the mind I would instantly fall into a deep sleep?" Repeat that question a number of times and hold the silent answer in mind with an expectation of sleep.

"What is the one thought that if it should arise in the mind I would instantly fall into a deep sleep?" Take note that this is the most important procedure in this entire book.

What is the thought that would send me to sleep?

Lying in bed ready for sleep ask yourself, "What do I want to do right now? Do I want to stay awake?" Wait for the answer, "No, I want to go to sleep." Continue, "What are the thoughts that I need to hold in mind in order for me to get to sleep and have a restful sleep and wake up in the morning feeling refreshed and energised?

What is the thought, that if I held it in mind, I would instantly relax into a deep sleep, such that I would have a peaceful sleep, a restful sleep, a rejuvenating sleep, a healthful sleep? What is the one thought that if it should arise in the mind I would instantly fall into a deep restful sleep? What is the thought, that if the unconscious mind just contemplated it would mean that my sleep becomes two to three times as deep?

It is all about the questions

What are the questions that I need to keep in mind such that I create a peaceful state of mind, such that I create good health, prosperity, success in business, and love and harmony in my relationships?

What type of thoughts would serve me right now? Being thoughts, doing thoughts, loving thoughts, playful thoughts? What is the context? Is this context about being or doing? What thoughts would be useful?

How do I direct my thoughts and dreams to create good health? To create my desired outcomes? The life that I desire? What thoughts do I need to support me towards self actualisation?

What are the thoughts I need to hold in mind such that at the end of the day I say to myself, "I had a great day. This was the best day of my life ever?" What are the thoughts that I need to hold in mind such that at the end of the week I look back and say to myself, "I had a great week. I had the time of my life. It was time well spent." What are the thoughts that I need to hold in mind such that at the end of the year I will say to myself, "This has been the best year of my life". What are the thoughts that I need to hold in mind such that at the end of my life I say to myself, This has been a life well worth having lived. I squeezed the juice from every moment. I accepted the challenges that life presented to me. I tapped into my inner resources. I set goals for myself and I took action such that I achieved results, such that I know at the deepest core of my being that I did the best that I possibly could.

In the evening and before going to sleep at night give suggestions to wake up the next morning feeling excited about the day. Give yourself something to look forwards to. Let it be a fantastic day, a million dollar day. Learn to look for the positive, the achievements, the successes, no matter how small they might be. Tomorrow will be a stepping stone towards evening greater successes.

How you talk to yourself (and others) will influence the meaning of the words. Our speech has three main distinctions: tempo, tonality and volume. The most important distinction is tonality. If you change the tonality then the entire meaning of the words can change in a single moment. Practise shifting the tonality from negative to positive.

Putting insomnia to sleep

What are the thoughts that I need to hold in mind such that I drift off to sleep right now, such that I have a restful sleep, a peaceful sleep, a healthful sleep, such that I have beautiful dreams, lovely dreams, healing dreams, such that when I wake up in the morning I feel refreshed, alert and energised, such that during the day I realise that the health problem must have miraculously disappeared during the night, such that now I feel so much more healthful, such that now I have so much more energy, such that now I find myself feeling so much more stronger, such that now I find myself taking action on my goals and achieving my goals with a growing sense of ease because this is what comes naturally to me.

So we ask, "Do these thoughts serve me right now? If not, then what thoughts would serve me? What are the thoughts that I need to hold in mind such that I find myself drifting off to sleep? What is the one thought that if it should arise in the mind I would instantly fall into a deep sleep?"

The pattern is:
"Do these thoughts serve me?"
"Is this what I want to be thinking about?"
If not, then:
"What thoughts would serve me right now?"

"What are the thoughts that I need to hold in mind such that... such that... such that... because..."

"What is the one thought that if it should arise in the mind I would instantly fall into a deep sleep?"

9

MEDITATION BASICS

This section provides a summary of meditation technique.

1. Witnessing is Essential
Witnessing means to see, to notice, to watch, to observe in a dispassionate manner. One learns to just see. One watches the thoughts like the movement of leaves on a tree. In most cases the movement of leaves in a tree, a bird across the sky, clouds across a sky, wind across a lake or the movement of people is not something that you think about. In most cases movement is something that you just notice. The art of noticing is what meditators refer to as witnessing or watching. Practise noticing the thoughts in your mind and you have the basis of every meditation technique.

2. Naughty Child Procedure
To help you understand how to witness your thoughts we use the analogy of a naughty child. Imagine that you are having a conversation with another adult. You have a two year old child in the room with you. When the two year old runs around the room making a noise you give her your attention. As long as you give her your full attention she stops still and remains quiet but

as soon as you start talking to your friend she is off and running again. Bring your attention back to her and she stops still and remains quiet. So as long as you give her your complete attention she will remain quiet.

Bring your critical awareness to the internal dialogue and it will quieten. Try it now. Start by becoming aware of your internal dialogue then bring your full attention to it. Don't think about the internal dialogue. Just be fully aware of it. What happens?

You should find that it becomes quieter, slows down, softens and moves further away. If you do it right the internal dialogue will disappear totally - for as long as you keep your awareness on it. This is a useful procedure if you are having difficulty getting to sleep as insomnia in many cases is just a result of rampant internal dialogue.

3. Mind Director Basics
We think in pictures, sounds and feelings. In each of those modalities there are sub distinctions known as submodalities. For example, internal dialogue will have a volume, tempo and tonality.

The following Mind Director technique can bring about profound results in a matter of moments. Lift up one of your arms and imagine that you have an imaginary control panel at your finger tips. It is like a graphic equaliser and has volume, tempo and tonality controls. Tune into your internal dialogue and turn down the volume. As you do this move your hand in the way that you would if you were to turn a dial. Don't think about turning the volume down, just turn it down, let it get smaller and smaller, smaller and smaller.

Now slow down the tempo. Use your hand to indicate that you are slowing down the tempo. Sometimes when you slow the speed of your self talk you may find a yawn coming to your throat. Once you have turned down the volume and slowed the tempo, soften the tonality. Let the tonality become softer and softer, let it become more friendly and more loving.

Turn down the volume, slow the tempo, soften the tonality and put the internal dialogue all the way out on the horizon, banishing all thoughts from the mind and entering into that space of silence that you enter into just before you drift off to sleep.

4. A Simple Sleep Meditation

When you are ready to go to sleep take your internal dialogue and put it out on the horizon. That is, imagine that the location of your internal dialogue is out on the horizon, and as long as it remains at that distance the mind becomes quiet. Bring your awareness to the silence.

Take any images that you have in your mind and turn

them to grey. I say grey, rather than black and white because even black and white can be too graphic, so just turn the imagery to grey. As you do so, you should notice that the images move further away and seem to lose their importance.

Turn down the internal dialogue and put it out on the horizon. Make the images grey and then put them out on the horizon. Notice where you naturally put the thoughts. The internal dialogue might go off to the left while the images go directly in front. In this way you put your mind out on the horizon. Keep your awareness on the silence; tell yourself to go to sleep, and remain a witness to the process.

5. Hypnosis

All meditation procedures rely upon hypnosis to a degree. To begin the meditator gives prestige to a teacher or to the source of the meditation procedure. This sets the frame. The meditator then sets an intention to achieve some outcome, such as entering into a no-mind state. The meditator practises a procedure which they believe will be helpful in attaining the desired outcome.

The meditator will need to access internal resources and may also draw upon external resources that support and enhance the meditation procedure. Throughout the entire process the meditator coaches themselves with a positive internal dialogue.

The temple may provide the context, the teacher may provide the prestige, the procedure itself may provide a means to progress towards the desired outcome but it is the quality of the conversation that the meditator has with their unconscious mind that determines the quality of the experience.

10

GLOSSARY

Awareness continuum

Is a procedure used by meditators in which you scan through the body, noticing if there is any pain, discomfort or tension there. The idea is not to become involved with the tension but to just be a dispassionate observer to it. One can scan the outside of the body or the inside, quickly or slowly.

Catalepsy

A condition characterised by muscular rigidity and a lack of response to an external stimuli. The limbs remain in whatever position they are placed. It occurs in epilepsy, schizophrenia and is a hypnotic phenomena. Arm catalepsy, where the arm of the subject floats in mid air, can be induced through hypnosis or it can occur spontaneously as a result of it. (*www.thefreedictionary.com/catalepsy*)

Catatonia

A condition characterized by either rigidity or extreme flexibility of the limbs. The terms 'catalepsy' and 'catatonia' seem to be used as synonyms in the context of hypnosis.

Eye closure

Means that the eye lids have closed. Eye catalepsy means that the eye lids are clamped shut. Sometimes the term 'eye closure' denotes 'eye catalepsy'. You need to get the meaning from the context in which it is used to make the distinction.

Eye catalepsy

See 'eye closure'.

Hypnosis

Hypnosis is the art of communicating with the unconscious mind. To explore consciousness one needs a concept of conscious and unconscious mind; to recognise the difference between willpower and imagination; to understand the process of suggestion and autosuggestion, and to have skills in ideosensory communication. With practice one learns how to give an autosuggestion with no self talk, and from being rather than intellect.

Ideomotor response

Ideo refers to mind. *Motor* refers to body. Ideomotor action is the tendency of thoughts to be translated into specific patterns of muscular activity. It is a communication from the unconscious mind expressed through body movement that is out of conscious control. Reflexes are examples of ideomotor action. Other examples are head nods and shakes, arm, finger and facial movements. In hypnosis the signals are known as ideomotor responses. By calibrating the signals for 'yes and no', a meaningful communication can be established with the unconscious mind.

Ideosensory response
An ideosensory response is an automatic response like the ideomotor response but it involves actions such as blushing or salivating at the thought of food.

Internal representation
A thought. More specifically a thought represented in one or more of the senses.

Meditation
Linguistically, meditation is classified as a noun but in fact meditation is a process of inquiry into the self. Meditation can have very different meanings depending upon the context. In the West, meditation is defined as an exercise in devotion or contemplation, sometimes on a religious or philosophical subject. Contemplation is an activity that uses the mind. In the East the purpose of meditation is to take you beyond the mind. Thinking is not something to be encouraged as the mind is seen as the root cause of all tensions, hence thinking is to be transcended.

Meditation is an effort to know the Witness. Once the content of the mind has been removed by witnessing there is no content for the mind to focus on and the

Witness turns back upon itself. *(Osho, The Fish in the Sea is not Thirsty. Ch 9 P 7.)*

Neuro Semantics

Developed by Dr L. Michael Hall, "Neuro Semantics is a model about how we create and embody meaning. And, of course, the way we create and embody meaning determines our sense of life and reality, our skills and competencies, and the quality of our experiences. Neuro-Semantics is a more scientific term for mind-body. As a field, Neuro-Semantics utilizes the Meta-States Model for understanding our unique kind of consciousness—self-reflexive consciousness. Neuro-Semantics is also an international association of men and women leading out in coaching and training regarding leadership, management, business, and self-actualization."

NLP

A model of psychology - a communication model - founded by Richard Bandler, John Grinder and Frank Pucelik in the early 1970's and developed with a host of co-developers over the next two decades. NLP is a modelling methodology that was initially applied to studying the excellence of Fritz Perls, Virginia Satir, and Milton Erickson. Most people think of NLP as the techniques when in fact they are the result of the modelling process.

Osho

Contemporary Zen Master, 11 December 1931 - 19 January 1990. Born in Kuchwada, a small village in the state of Madhya Pradesh, central India. Becomes enlightened at the age of twenty-one, while majoring in philosophy at D.N. Jain college in Jabalpur. 1957-1966 University Professor and Public Speaker. 1966 onwards devotes himself to raising human consciousness. Addresses gatherings of 20,000 - 50,000. For a complete biography visit www.otoons.com/osho/

Pendulum

A hypnosis pendulum (a marble on a piece of string) employs an ideomotor response from the unconscious mind and can be calibrated to give a rapid and precise signal for 'yes and no', and 'to what degree'.

Peripheral sensing

Utilising the peripheral aspects of the sense organs rather than focussing in. For example, in the visual modality you can concentrate on what is in the direct field of vision or relax into an awareness of what is in the periphery. In the auditory modality you can concentrate on one sound or just be aware of the sounds around you that move into and out of your awareness. When you bring peripheral sensing to one modality it tends to relax you into peripheral sensing in the others too.

Submodalities

Sub distinctions within the visual, auditory, kinaesthetic, olfactory and gustatory senses. Examples of visual submodalities: colour, black and white, movie, still, size, brightness. Examples of auditory submodalities: volume, tonality and tempo. Examples of kinaesthetic submodalities: location, sensation, temperature, pressure, tension, movement and size.

When you think of a visual memory are you looking out of your own eyes and seeing yourself in the memory? Where is the image located in respect of the body? Directly in front, above, below, behind, to the left or right side, and so on? If you hear a voice in your mind where is the location of the voice? What is the volume, tonality and tempo? If you experience a feeling, then what is the location, temperature, size, tension, strength and so on? When you change submodalities in one channel it will affect submodalities in another channel due to synaesthesia in the brain.

Trance state

A trance is an altered state of consciousness. In common usage it refers to losing conscious awareness of one's surrounding and entering a daydream or waking sleep state. At the extremes one may enter a trance through ecstatic dance or by sitting with closed eyes in meditation.

Universal love and healing energy

The concept of universal energy holds that a range of energies are freely available to everyone to tap into. All one need do is open their mind and heart to the energy and then channel it to a specific part of the mind or body for a desired outcome. Typical universal energies are 'love and healing' and 'power and strength.

IMAGE PERMISSIONS

Cover image: Night Scape ID: 416240 © Scott Rothstein | Dreamstime.com

ACKNOWLEDGMENTS

To Osho for everything.

Thank you to the NLP community for the *'Drug of Choice'* procedure. I think it may have been originally developed by Richard Bandler.

Thank you to Davel Elman for his *'Relax the muscles around the eyes and dropping down through the levels'* trance induction procedure.

REFERENCES

All efforts have been made to correctly reference sources of information. If there has been an oversight please contact Abby Eagle from www.abbyeagle.com.

Abby Eagle's diary notes can be found at http://www.abbyeagle.com/blog/

BIBLIOGRAPHY

Elman, Dave. *Hypnotherapy.* Westwood Publishing Co. Glendale, CA, USA 1964.

Hall, Michael. *Accessing Personal Genius* DVD set.

Osho. *The Tantra Vision, Vol 1* pages 5-20. Osho Foundation International.

ABOUT THE AUTHOR

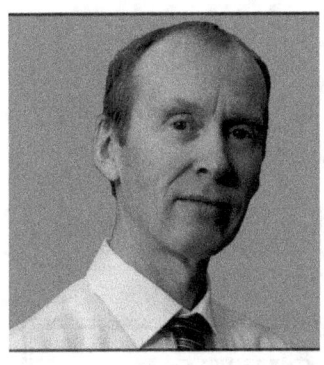

Abby Eagle spent 12 years working as a laboratory technician / photographer in the Department of Botany at the University of Western Australia (1972-1984) before backpacking across Indonesia. He then travelled to the USA to visit the Osho commune in Oregon that later became a benchmark for land reclamation, and has spent some time in India and Malaysia. Abby has a Diploma in Applied Science (Biology); is a Master Practitioner of NLP, Ericksonian Hypnosis and Time-Line Therapy™; is a certified Neuro Semantic Meta Coach, and has 30 years experience in the personal growth field and eastern meditative techniques. His genius is creativity; his passion is film making and his purpose is to wake people up. Abby Eagle lives on the Gold Coast, Queensland, Australia.

Contact Abby Eagle
PO Box 902, Palm Beach, Qld 4221 Australia.
Website: www.abbyeagle.com
Email: abbyeagle@rejoiceinlife.com
Facebook: https://www.facebook.com/abbyeagle

FIND ABBY EAGLE

WWW.ABBYEAGLE.COM

FACEBOOK

LINKEDIN

YOUTUBE

SPECIAL OFFER
50% OFF COUPON

TYT9UNOIHU229

Buy the "Put Insomnia To Sleep" package from www.abbyeagle.com so that you can download and listen to the mp3 audio files.

VISIT
www.abbyeagle.com/shoppingcart/products/Put-insomnia-to-sleep.html

---

Appendix